RENAL DIET COOKBOOK FOR BEGINNERS

An ultimate guide to renal eating Wellness: Savoring Life with Flavorful Journey through Culinary Bliss." Tasty recipes for a healthy and vibrant you.

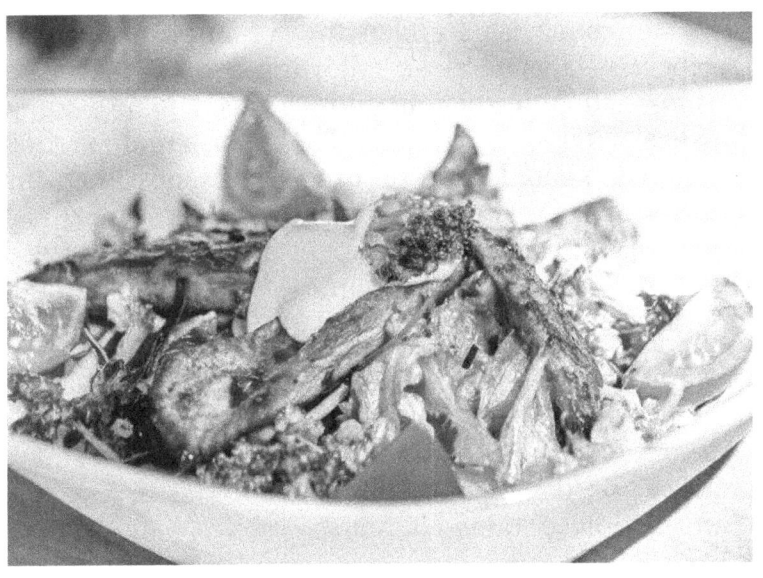

BRENDA.M. SMITH

Copyright © 2024 BY BRENDA.M. SMITH

This cookbook is intended to give information and recipes specific to those following a renal diet. The author and publisher are not engaged in providing medical advice or services. The information in this cookbook should not be used as a substitute for professional medical care or guidance. Consult a certified healthcare practitioner for tailored advice based on your health situation.

While every effort has been made to ensure the accuracy and completeness of the information presented in this cookbook, the author and publisher assume no responsibility for errors or omissions, misuse, or damages resulting from the use of the information contained herein.

TABLE OF CONTENT

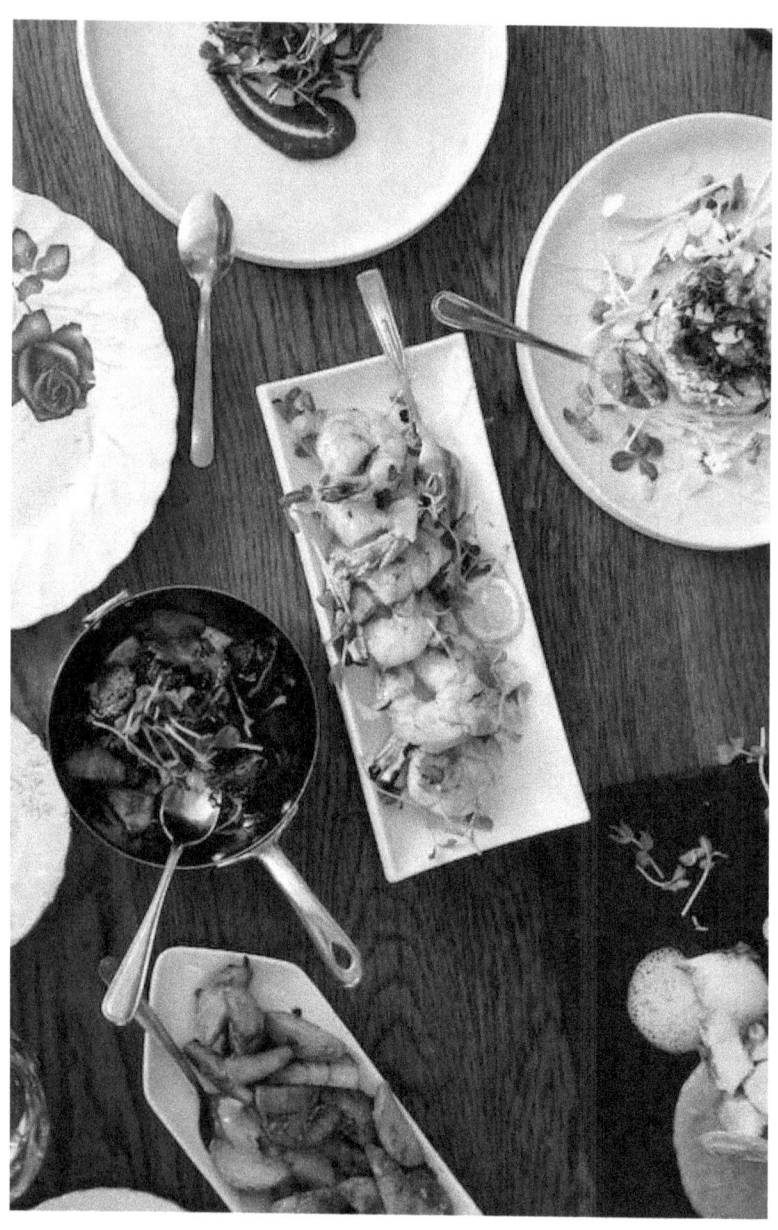

INTRODUCTION

Susan discovered a newfound passion for cooking when her father's kidney health required dietary adjustments. Frustrated by limited recipes, she stumbled upon a renal cookbook at the local library. With cautious enthusiasm, she delved into its pages, meticulously following its kidney-friendly guidelines.

A transformation occurred in her kitchen as she chopped, stirred, and baked her way through its recipes. Dull meals turned into vibrant culinary creations bursting with flavor and vitality. Each dish not only nourished but also lifted her father's spirits.

Their dining table became a stage for new gastronomic wonders, sparking joyous conversations and heartfelt connections. Empowered by the cookbook's guidance, Susan's family bonded over delightful meals that supported her father's health and enriched their shared experiences. The renal cookbook evolved beyond a guide—it became a beacon of hope, turning meals into moments of love and wellness.

The Kidney

The kidneys are vital organs in the human body that filter waste and excess blood fluids to form urine. They are crucial in maintaining overall fluid balance, regulating electrolytes, and producing hormones that control blood pressure, red blood cell production, and bone health. Each person typically has two kidneys on either side of the spine, just below the rib cage. The kidneys are essential for maintaining the body's overall health and function.

Importance of the kidney to the general health.

Filtration of Waste: The kidneys filter waste products, excess salts, and toxins from the blood, preventing a buildup of harmful substances in the body. These waste products are then excreted as urine.

Regulation of Fluid Balance: They help maintain the body's fluid balance by adjusting the amount of water excreted as urine based on hydration levels and other bodily needs.

Blood Pressure Regulation: Kidneys play a crucial role in regulating blood pressure by controlling the balance of sodium, potassium, and other electrolytes in the blood.

Red Blood Cell Production: They produce a hormone called erythropoietin, which stimulates the bone marrow to produce red blood cells. Red blood cells carry oxygen to tissues and organs.

Acid-Base Balance: Kidneys help regulate the body's pH levels by controlling the levels of acids and bases in the blood.

Activation of Vitamin D: They contribute to the activation of vitamin D, which is essential for calcium absorption and bone health.

Hormone Production: Apart from erythropoietin, kidneys produce other hormones involved in various bodily functions, including regulating blood pressure (renin) and assisting in red blood cell production (erythropoietin).

CHAPTER 1: THE RENAL DIET

The renal diet is a customized eating regimen that promotes kidney health and helps those with kidney disease. This diet focuses on managing the consumption of key nutrients such as sodium, potassium, phosphorus, and protein to regulate the workload of the kidneys and maintain optimal function. The renal diet tries to relieve stress on the kidneys, control fluid balance, and minimize waste product buildup in the circulation by carefully monitoring these factors. This dietary strategy is critical in sustaining overall kidney function and increasing the quality of life for those who have renal problems.

Nutritional Guidelines of the renal health.

Protein: proteins are large, complex molecules of smaller units called amino acids. They are crucial for various functions in the body, such as building and repairing tissues, supporting immune function, producing enzymes and hormones, and serving as a source of energy.

In terms of renal health, proteins play a significant role. As part of the renal system, the kidneys help filter waste products and excess substances, including byproducts from protein metabolism. When proteins are broken down in the body, urea produces one of the waste products. Healthy kidneys efficiently filter urea and other waste products out of the blood, then excreted as urine. However, in individuals with kidney problems or reduced kidney function, properly filtering waste, including urea and other byproducts of protein metabolism, can be compromised. This can lead to a buildup of these substances in the blood, causing complications and contributing to further kidney damage. Managing protein intake might be crucial for individuals with kidney disease or impaired renal function.

A doctor or a renal dietitian might recommend controlling the amount of protein consumed to lessen the strain on the kidneys. This could involve adjusting the type and quantity of protein in the diet to help manage kidney function and reduce the buildup of waste products. Balancing protein intake while considering individual health conditions is essential for optimal renal health.

Sodium:

Sodium is an electrolyte and mineral that is essential for many body activities. It aids in maintaining balance, neuron function, and muscle contractions. However, sodium is more commonly found in nature as a compound, such as sodium chloride (table salt) or sodium bicarbonate (baking soda).

Excess salt consumption, on the other hand, can cause health problems, particularly in the kidneys.

The kidneys are important in controlling salt levels in the body. They filter the blood to eliminate waste and excess chemicals such as salt. When there is an excess of salt in the circulation, the kidneys must work harder to eliminate it through urine. High salt consumption can strain the kidneys over time, potentially leading to issues such as:

High Blood Pressure: Because sodium draws water, the blood in the circulation increases. This can raise blood pressure, burdening the kidneys over time. High blood pressure can harm the kidneys and raise the risk of renal disease.

Kidney Stones: Excess salt can cause increased calcium levels in the urine, which can contribute to the production of kidney stones. These stones can cause excruciating pain and impair kidney function.

Kidney Disease: Long-term excessive salt consumption and high blood pressure can harm the kidneys. This damage can proceed to chronic kidney disease, impairing the kidneys' capacity to function and leading to consequences including fluid retention and electrolyte abnormalities.

Examples of dietary sodium sources include:

The most well-known source of sodium is **table salt** (Sodium Chloride). It is frequently used in cooking and added to processed goods to add taste and preserve them.

Processed Foods: To improve taste and extend shelf life, many processed and packaged foods include high levels of salt. Examples include Canned soups, processed meats (such as bacon and ham), snack foods, and fast food products.

Natural Sources: Some naturally occurring salt may be found in some crops (celery, beets), dairy products, and ter.

Potassium: Potassium is a mineral and electrolyte that is essential for many body activities such as muscle contractions, neuron function, fluid balance, and heart rhythm. It is a necessary nutrient for the body to function correctly. Potassium is connected to renal health because of its involvement in electrolyte balance and kidney functions such as fluid balance, blood pressure control, and kidney diseases however, Potassium levels can become too high (hyperkalemia) in people with impaired kidney function or certain medical disorders, such as chronic kidney disease. In such circumstances, the kidneys may struggle to eliminate extra potassium, potentially leading to irregular heartbeat and renal Health weakness.

Controlling potassium consumption is critical for people who have renal problems. A healthcare physician or a qualified dietitian may advise you on how to maintain adequate potassium levels through food, especially if you have renal disease. They may advise reducing potassium consumption or utilizing certain cooking methods to minimize potassium levels in certain meals. Individuals with renal difficulties must have their potassium levels checked regularly to avoid consequences.

Phosphorus: Phosphorus is a mineral in the body in the form of phosphate. It is essential for several body activities, including bone health, energy generation, and cell membrane modulation.

Managing phosphorus consumption is critical for those with renal problems, particularly those with impaired kidney function or CKD. Controlling phosphorus levels with diet, phosphate binders, and regular renal care helps to avoid issues associated with excessive phosphorus levels.

Dairy products, meat, fish, nuts, seeds, whole grains, and some processed meals are high in phosphorus. To assist in controlling phosphorus levels and minimize strain on the kidneys in situations of renal disease, healthcare practitioners frequently recommend restricting high-phosphorus diets. For people with renal disease, consulting with a healthcare expert or a trained dietitian for advice on a proper diet and phosphorus consumption is critical.

Fluids intake: Fluid consumption is essential for maintaining healthy kidneys and good renal function. The kidneys filter waste materials and excess fluids from the blood to make urine, which maintains the body's water and electrolyte balance.

Maintaining adequate hydration is critical for good kidney function. It aids the kidneys in efficiently filtering waste and toxins from the blood. When you're well-hydrated, your body has adequate fluid to clear waste materials efficiently through urine.

IMPORTANCE OF FLUID INTAKE

Preventing Kidney Stones: Drinking enough fluids, especially water, dilutes chemicals in the urine, making minerals and salts less prone to crystallize and create kidney stones. Dehydration can cause concentrated urine, which increases the likelihood of stone development.

Blood Pressure Regulation: Adequate hydration aids in the maintenance of blood volume, which impacts blood pressure regulation. Dehydration can encourage the kidneys to save water, resulting in elevated blood pressure. This can put a load on the kidneys and cardiovascular system over time.

Fluid Balance and Electrolytes: Fluid intake is intimately linked to electrolyte balance, such as sodium, potassium, and chloride. Hydration is important for kidney health and general physiological processes because it maintains a balance between fluid intake and electrolyte levels. Excess fluid consumption beyond the body's demands, on the other hand, can strain the kidneys, especially in people with renal problems or impaired kidney function. In such circumstances, the kidneys may struggle to adequately absorb and discharge excess fluids, resulting in fluid retention and possible problems.

Inadequate fluid intake, which causes dehydration, can potentially affect the kidneys. Dehydration lowers the amount of blood going through the kidneys, reducing their ability to adequately filter waste and toxins.

Fluid intake must be balanced. Individuals differ in age, climate, physical activity level, and general health. Staying hydrated by drinking water and ingesting fluids from diverse sources such as fruits, vegetables, and soups will help kidney health. Monitoring urine color (from light yellow to clear) and reacting to thirst signals are both important markers of enough water for optimal kidney health. Fluid intake guidelines from healthcare providers are critical for persons with unique renal disorders to preserve kidney function and general well-being.

CHAPTER 2: BREAKFAST RECIPES

Egg White Omelets with Vegetables

INGREDIENTS   **2 servings**

4 eggs white

¼ cup fresh spinach

1 garlic clove minced

½ cup bell pepper chopped

 onion chopped

½ teaspoon black pepper

2 tbsp. oil (coconut, olive, or avocado oil)

Spring onion

½ teaspoon ground black pepper

Procedure

- Beat eggs with pepper until light and fluffy.
- Sauté the bell peppers, spinach, and onions until slightly softened
- In a large skillet, heat the oil over medium heat.
- Pour the egg into the skillet and add the garlic and onions.
- Add cooked vegetables
- Cook until set and fold.

Chia Seed Pudding

INGREDIENTS   **1 servings**

¼ cup chia seeds

1 cup plant-based milk (coconut milk /almond milk)

1 tsp. vanilla extract

½ Tbsp. Maple syrup or honey (optional)

1/4 tsp. cinnamon

Sliced fruit for topping (berries or banana)

Procedure

- Mix chia seeds with coconut milk, vanilla extract, and a touch of maple syrup if using
- Stir well and refrigerate for at least two hours until it thickens or refrigerate overnight
- top with low-potassium fruits

Avocado toast

INGREDIENTS   **4 slices of toast**

4 slices of gluten-free bread

1 avocado mashed or sliced

2 pinch red pepper flakes

2 pinch of sea salt

a squeeze of fresh lemon or lime (opt)

procedure

- Toast 4 bread
- Place mashed or sliced avocado on the bread
- Add a sprinkle of red pepper flakes or sea salt to taste.

Egg and Veggie Muffin Cups

INGREDIENTS   **6 servings**

½ cup vegetables diced small or shredded (carrot, yellow squash, red pepper)

1 /2 teaspoon oil

4 eggs

1 tablespoon fresh herbs (dill, basil, and parsley)

2 stalks green onion and white thinly sliced

1 teaspoon mayonnaise

Brie cheese (small slices) Optional

1 teaspoon lemon zest to taste

procedure

• In a mixing dish, combine the eggs and mayonnaise, and add herbs and sliced green onions.

• Stir in the cooked veggies.

• Divide the batter among 6 muffin cups. (Silicon muffin or a 9x9 dish) add a little piece of brie if using. Bake at 350°F for 20-25 minutes, or until the center of each muffin is set. Top each muffin with a sprinkling of lemon zest.

Tofu veggie scramble

INGREDIENTS   **1 serving**

½ cup firm or extra firm tofu crumbled

1 tablespoons olive oil

1 onion peeled and finely diced

1 tomatoes (opt)

1 cloves garlic peeled and minced (opt)

¼ cup diced bell pepper

 cauliflower, / spinach cut into small florets

¼ teaspoon turmeric

1 tablespoons nutritional yeast

¼ teaspoon black pepper

Pinch of salt / add to first

Procedure

- Over medium heat, heat olive oil in a skillet, once heated, add the diced onion, bell peppers, cauliflower/spinach, and garlic if using until softens.
- Add crumbled tofu, sprinkle the yeast if using, and add black pepper, salt, and turmeric.

- Cook until the cauliflower/spinach is soft, with the crumbled tofu or has heated through
- Serve warm

Rice Cake with Almond Butter and Berries

INGREDIENTS

1 Rice cake,

I tsp almond butter,

 Berries

Sweetener (optional)

procedure

- spread the almond butter on the rice cake
- enjoy with any low-potassium berries of your choice
- sprinkle either honey or maple syrup

Apples cinnamon overnight oat

INGREDIENTS:

1/2 cup rolled oats

½ cup unsweetened almond milk

 diced apples, (to your taste)

1 tsp chopped almond

½ tablespoon cinnamon

1 /2 tbsp Flax seed (optional)

Procedure:

- in a bowl or jar mix the milk and the oat
- add chopped almond, diced apple, cinnamon, and flax seed and mix well.
- cover and leave in the refrigerator overnight
- in the morning enjoy either cold or warm.

Breakfast burrito

INGREDIENT   **1 serving**

1 whole wheat tortilla, burrito size

2 eggs,

¼ cup low-sodium cooked black beans,

tablespoon tomatoes diced

2 tablespoons diced onions

1/2 teaspoon ground cumin

hot pepper sauce

Procedure

- Oil the skillet and heat over medium heat
- In a bowl, beat the egg, add the ground cumin, and hot pepper sauce, and scramble
- Add the diced tomatoes, onions, and the black bean in the egg to warm

- Heat tortillas in another skillet or an oven for some seconds
- Fill the tortilla with scrambled egg and roll it up.

NOTE: you can enjoy by adding bell peppers, vegetables of your choice, and cheese.

Veggie Breakfast Skillet

INGREDIENTS   **1 serving**

1/2 cup diced potatoes

2 tablespoons chopped onions

¼ cup spinach

2 tablespoons diced tomatoes

¼ cup chopped bell peppers

¼ teaspoon paprika

1 teaspoon olive oil

procedure

- In medium heat, heat oil in a skillet
- Add diced potatoes and cook until slightly golden.
- Stir onions, tomatoes, spinach, bell peppers, and paprika.
- Cook until vegetables are tender.

Sweet potato hash

INGREDIENTS   **1 serve**

1 cup diced sweet potatoes,

One small onions diced

1 tsp olive oil

Small red bell pepper

Small green bell pepper

½ tablespoon paprika

Black pepper (sprinkle)

procedure

- Slice the sweet potatoes and cook on low heat
- In a skillet, fry the chopped onions, and bell peppers until tender
- Add the boiled potatoes and stir
- Add paprika and sprinkle black pepper

French toast

INGREDIENTS

2 slices bread,

1 egg,

½ cup almond milk,

½ tsp vanilla extract

Pinch of ground cloves

Pinch of ground cinnamon

Procedure

- Beat the egg, mix the milk, vanilla extract, cinnamon, cloves and mix thoroughly
- Grease the skimmer with olive oil or unsalted butter
- Dip the bread in the mixture and cook until golden brown on each side

Buckwheat Porridge

INGREDIENTS

¼ cup buckwheat groats,

1 cup almond milk

1 tbsp honey, / maple syrup

chopped nuts

fruits (optional) to garnish

½ tsp ground cinnamon

vanilla extract (a few drops)

water

procedure

- Rinse the buckwheat and on boiling water with low heat, pour the buckwheat and stir until the water is absorbed and the buckwheat is tender

- Add the milk and stir
- Add the sweetener, stir and dish
- Add your nuts and fruits

Smoked Salmon Bagel

INGREDIENTS

1 whole-grain bagel, cut and toasted

2 oz. smoked salmon

2 tbsp. low-fat cream cheese

Cucumber

red onion, thinly sliced (optional)

Garnish with fresh dill

Arugula leaves (to content)

Procedure

- Cream cheese should be spread on the toasted bagel halves.
- Place the smoked salmon on top.
- If desired, garnish with cucumber and red onion slices.
- Add the arugula and Serve open-faced with fresh dill garnish.

NOTE: you can add egg, and scallions or serve with any vegetable of your choice.

Quinoa Breakfast Bowl:

INGREDIENTS   2 serve

1/2 cup quinoa

1/4 cup strawberries, sliced

Blueberries (desired)

2 tbsp. almonds, chopped or (hazelnut, walnut)

1 teaspoon honey /maple syrup

Procedure

- Add water to the quinoa in a medium saucepan and cook on a low heat /cook according to package instructions.
- Layer cooked quinoa, strawberries, blueberries, and almonds in a bowl.
- Serve with honey drizzled over top.

Pancakes

INGREDIENTS

1 cup all-purpose flour

½ tsp. baking soda

½ tsp cream of tartar(opt)

1 tsp sugar

½ tsp salt

1 cup almond milk/any low-fat milk

1 tbsp. canola oil

1 egg (optional)

½ tablespoon vinegar

Procedure

- Make sour milk by adding the vinegar to be left for a few minutes if using.
- In a mixing basin, combine the flour, sugar, cream of tartar (opt), baking soda, and salt.
- Whisk in the almond milk and oil gradually until smooth.
- If using egg, beat egg to fluffy and add the milk and oil mixed
- Mix the dry ingredients and mix till smooth
- To prepare pancakes, heat a nonstick pan over medium heat and pour batter into the pan.
- Cook until surface bubbles appear, then turn and cook until golden brown.
- Serve with a small quantity of maple syrup or honey.

Note: you can use almond flour or buckwheat flour to make pancakes following the same procedure

Greek yogurt parfait with seeds

INGREDIENTS:

1 cup Greek yogurt

2 tablespoons chia seeds

2 tablespoons pumpkin seeds

1/4 cup sliced strawberries/raspberries

1 teaspoon vanilla extract (optional)

1 tablespoon honey or sweetener (optional)

Procedure

- Mix the yogurt with vanilla extract if using and layer in a glass or bowl, layer Greek yogurt, chia seeds, pumpkin seeds, and sliced strawberries.
- Repeat layers as desired.
- Drizzle with honey if using and serve chilled.

Egg White and Veggie Scramble:

INGREDIENTS: **2 servings**

3 egg whites

I cup fresh spinach

¼ cup cauliflower/mushroom

¼ cup diced zucchini (optional)

Bell peppers

2 tablespoons of finely chopped onions

1 tsp olive oil

salt and black pepper.

Spring onion for garnish (optional)

procedure

- In a skillet over medium heat, warm the olive oil.

- Onions, mushrooms, bell peppers spinach, and zucchini should be sautéed until soft.

- Season the skillet with salt and pepper and add the egg whites.

- Until the eggs are set, cook and stir them.

Berries and Millet Porridge

INGREDIENTS: **2 servings**

½ cup millet

½ cup of almond milk or any plant-based milk

¼ cup mixed berries, including blackberries and raspberries

2 tablespoons of chopped nuts (almonds, walnuts)

1 tablespoon of sweetener

½ tablespoon ground cinnamon (optional)

water

procedure

- After rinsing, put the millet in a saucepan with water and cinnamon if using.

- After bringing it to a boil, lower the heat, and simmer the millet for 15-20 minutes, or until it becomes soft.

- After turning off the heat, leave it alone for a while.

- Serve in bowls and garnish with honey, almonds, or mixed berries, if desired.

Low-Potassium Breakfast Burrito Bowl

INGREDIENTS: **1 servings**

½ cup cooked brown rice

¼ cup black beans (rinsed and drained)

¼ cup diced tomatoes

2 tablespoons diced onions

2 tablespoons chopped cilantro

¼ avocado, sliced (optional)

Lime wedges for garnish

1 full egg scrambled (optional)

procedure:

- In a bowl, layer brown rice, black beans, tomatoes, onions, and cilantro.

- Layer the egg if using

- Top with avocado slices if using and serve with lime wedges.

Veggie Breakfast Casserole

INGREDIENTS: **2-3 servings**

4 eggs

½ cup chopped spinach

½ cup diced bell peppers

½   onions diced

½ cup low-fat shredded cheese

Salt and black pepper to taste

Chopped parsley for garnish (optional)

procedure

- Set oven temperature to 175°C/350°F.

- In a bowl, whisk eggs and add pepper and salt to taste.

- Add bell peppers, onions, spinach, and half of the cheese

- Transfer the mixture to a baking dish that has been oiled.

- Top with the remaining cheese sprinkled on and the parsley if using

- Bake the eggs for 20 to 25 minutes, or until set.

Cottage Cheese Pancakes

INGREDIENTS: **1-2 servings**

1 cup low-fat cottage cheese

2 whole eggs or 3 egg white

1/4 cup whole wheat flour

1/2 teaspoon baking powder

1 teaspoon vanilla extract

Cooking spray

To prepare,

- blend cottage cheese, eggs, flour, baking powder, and vanilla extract until a smooth consistency is achieved.

- Coat a nonstick pan with cooking spray and heat it over medium heat.

- To prepare pancakes, pour batter into the pan. After bubbling, turn, and continue cooking until golden brown.

Breakfast Wrap with Turkey and Spinach

INGREDIENTS: **1-2 servings**

1 whole-grain wrap

2 slices low-sodium turkey breast

¼ cup chopped spinach

½ onions diced

Bell peppers

1 tablespoon low-fat cream cheese

procedure

- Slice turkey into tiny pieces and sauté. Sauté onion, bell peppers
- Spread the wrap on a flat surface
- Spread cream cheese over the wrap.
- Layer turkey slices, peppers, and chopped spinach in the center
- Roll it up tightly, slice it in half, and serve.

Peanut Butter and Banana Toast

INGREDIENTS: 1 serve

1 slice of whole-grain bread

1 tablespoon natural peanut butter

½ banana, sliced

procedure:

- Toast the bread until golden brown.
- Spread peanut butter on the toast.
- Top with banana slices and serve.

Fruit Salad with Mint-Lime Dressing

INGREDIENTS:

1 cup mixed fruits (melon, pineapple, seedless grapes berries)

½ tablespoon freshly squeezed lime juice

1 teaspoon honey

Fresh mint leaves for garnish

procedure

- Cut fruits into bite-sized pieces and place in a bowl.
- In a small bowl, mix lime juice and honey to create the dressing.
- Drizzle the dressing over the fruits and toss gently.
- Garnish with fresh mint leaves and serve.

Low-Sodium Breakfast Sausage Patties

INGREDIENTS: **2-3 (2 patties per serving)**

½ pound lean ground turkey

½ teaspoon sage

½ teaspoon thyme

¼ teaspoon black pepper

¼ teaspoon garlic powder

procedure

- In a bowl, mix ground turkey with sage, thyme, black pepper, and garlic powder.

- Form into small patties.

- Heat a non-stick skillet over medium heat and cook patties until browned and cooked through.

- Enjoy with any toppings of your choice (fruits, vegetables, milk bun)

CHAPTER 3: LUNCH RECIPES

Grilled Lemon Herb Chicken

INGREDIENTS: **4 servings**

4 boneless, skinless chicken breasts

2 tablespoons olive oil

2 cloves garlic, minced

1 teaspoon dried thyme

1 teaspoon dried rosemary

2 tablespoons lemon juice

½ teaspoon ground black pepper

Lemon wedges(optional)

procedure

- Mix olive oil, pepper, garlic, thyme, rosemary, and lemon juice.

- Marinate chicken in the mixture for 30 minutes.

- Grill chicken until fully cooked.

- Serve with a side of steamed vegetables and brown rice.

Quinoa Salad

INGREDIENTS: **3-4 servings**

1 cup quinoa, cooked

1 seedless cucumber, diced

1 red bell pepper, chopped

¼ cup chopped parsley

2 tablespoons olive oil

2 tablespoons lemon juice

3 spring onion chopped

4 cherry tomatoes diced (optional)

Procedure

- Mix cooked quinoa with cucumber, bell pepper, onion, tomatoes and parsley.

- Add olive oil and lemon juice and toss well.

- Serve on a bowl or spoon in lettuce cups

Note: you can cook the quinoa with vegetable broth

Vegetable Stir-Fry

INGREDIENTS: **2-3 servings**

2 cups mixed vegetables (broccoli or mushroom, snap peas, celery)

2 tablespoons olive oil

2 cloves garlic, minced

1 medium red bell pepper

1 medium green bell pepper

4 cherry tomatoes (optional)

½ small onion

½ teaspoon dried oregano

¼ teaspoon ground pepper

1 tablespoon low-sodium soy sauce

procedure

- Heat oil in a large skillet, add mushroom, celery bell peppers, oregano, onion, and snap peas until tender

- Add pepper, tomatoes, soy sauce and stir

- Serve on brown rice or quinoa

Roasted Vegetable Pasta (primavera)

INGREDIENTS: **3 servings**

8 oz whole wheat pasta

2 cups mixed roasted vegetables (bell peppers, cherry tomatoes, squash, carrot, broccoli)

2 tablespoons olive oil

2 cloves garlic, minced

1/4 cup grated Parmesan cheese

1 tablespoon of all-purpose flour

2 tablespoons half-and-half creamer (optional

1 cup low-sodium chicken broth (optional)

Procedure

- Cook pasta according to package instructions without salt. Drain and set aside.
- Roast or cook the vegetables until tender
- In a pan, heat olive oil, add garlic, and sauté.
- Pour in the chicken stock and cook on a low heat.
- Add the all-purpose flour and stir to avoid clumps, add half and half and simmer.
- Toss in roasted vegetables and cooked pasta. Sprinkle with Parmesan cheese.

Note: this recipe can be enjoyed without cream, stock, and, flour by frying your garlic with oil, adding the pasta, vegetables and cook, and finally adding the cheese

Tuna Salad Lettuce Wraps

INGREDIENTS: **2 -3 servings**

2 cans tuna in water, drained (8 ounces)

¼ cup plain Greek yogurt or mayonnaise

1 celery stalk, diced

1 tablespoon lemon juice

Lettuce leaves for wrapping

fresh dill for toppings

¼ teaspoon granulated sugar (optional)

½ onion (optional)

procedure

- In a bowl, mix tuna, Greek yogurt, celery, onion, sugar if using, and lemon juice.

- Spoon tuna salad onto lettuce leaves, garnish with fresh sliced dill, and, fold

- Or scoop in a whole-grain wrap and enjoy

Chicken and Vegetable Brown Rice

INGREDIENTS: **3 servings**

2 cups brown rice cooked

2 chicken breasts, cooked and shredded

1 ½ cup mixed vegetables (peas, carrots, corn, bell peppers, broccoli or mushroom)

1 clove minced garlic (optional)

½ onion cut into small wedges

2 tablespoons low-sodium soy sauce

1 tablespoon sesame oil

Procedure

- In a pan, combine cooked brown rice, shredded chicken, and mixed vegetables. Stir in soy sauce and sesame oil. Cook for 5-7 minutes until heated through.

OR

- Sauté onion, and garlic in oil, add the shredded chicken, vegetables, and soy sauce, and serve over the cooked brown rice

Eggplant and Tomato Bake

INGREDIENTS: **4 servings**

2 eggplants, sliced

4 tomatoes, sliced

1 cup grated Parmesan cheese

1 cup breadcrumbs (optional)

2 tablespoons olive oil

2 cloves garlic, minced

1 ½ teaspoon oregano for garnish

Procedure

- Preheat oven to 375°F (190°C). Grease a baking dish.

- Layer eggplant and tomato slices in the dish. Sprinkle with garlic and breadcrumbs if using.

- Drizzle with olive oil, top with Parmesan cheese, and Bake for 25-30 minutes until vegetables are tender and cheese is golden.

chicken and Vegetable Skewers

INGREDIENTS: **4 servings**

1-pound boneless, skinless chicken thigh cut into chunks (turkey can also do)

1 tablespoon peach jam liquify

2 bell peppers, cut into squares

1 zucchini, sliced

2 tablespoons olive oil

1 medium onion

1 medium yellow summer squash

1 teaspoon paprika

Pinch of dried ground sage

Salt and pepper to taste

Procedure

- Make the marinade by mixing the olive oil, peach jam, paprika, sage, salt, and pepper and stirring until blended.
- Add some marinade to the chicken and refrigerate to marinate.

- Place the already bite-sized vegetable in a bowl and add the reserved marinade, stir to coat the vegetables

- Preheat the grill or broiler and Thread chicken, bell peppers, onion, and zucchini onto skewers.

- Grill for 10-15 minutes covered and turn occasionally to cook evenly

Lentil Soup

INGREDIENTS: 4 servings

1 cup dried lentils

4 cups low-sodium chicken stock /vegetable broth

I tablespoon of extra-virgin olive oil

1 onion, chopped

2 carrots, diced

2 celery stalks, chopped

2 cloves garlic, minced

1 teaspoon dried thyme (optional)

Ground pepper to taste

2 tablespoons lemon juice

1 cup chard leave /spinach

procedure

- In a medium pot, heat the oil over medium heat and sauté onion and minced garlic.

- Add the lentils, carrot, celery, thyme if using, and broth, and bring to a boil for about 12- 15 minutes.

- Add the chard or spinach, cook for 2-3 minutes until wilted and

- Season with lemon juice and pepper and serve

Baked Salmon with Herbs

INGREDIENTS: 4 servings

4 salmon fillets

2 tablespoons chopped fresh dill

1 tablespoon olive oil

1 lemon, juice and zest

2 garlic cloves minced

Salt and pepper to taste

Serve alongside roasted asparagus, brown rice, or salad.

Procedure

- Preheat oven to 375°F (190°C). on a baking sheet place the salmon filets.

- Rub fillets with olive oil, sprinkle with salt, pepper, fresh lemon juice, and zest, add the fresh dill, and garlic, and top with sliced lemon.

- Bake for 12-15 minutes until salmon flakes easily with a fork.

Cauliflower Rice Stir-Fry

INGREDIENTS: **4 servings**

1 head cauliflower, grated into rice-like texture

1 cup chopped mixed vegetables (bell peppers, carrots, peas)

2 cloves garlic, minced

1 medium onion diced

½ cup purple cabbage (optional)

2 tablespoons low-sodium soy sauce

1 tablespoon sesame oil

2 stalks green onions or spring onion chopped

Salt and pepper to taste

Procedure

- Heat sesame oil in a skillet, add garlic, and onion and stir for a minute.

- Add cauliflower rice and mixed vegetables. Cook until vegetables are tender.

- Add soy sauce, green onions, salt, and pepper, and mix well.

Mushroom and Spinach Frittata

INGREDIENTS: **4-6 servings**

8 eggs

1 cup sliced mushrooms

2 cups fresh spinach

1 teaspoon fresh dried dill

½ cup diced onion

½ cup shredded low-fat cheese

1 tablespoon olive oil

1 clove garlic minced

A pinch of thyme

¼ tablespoon black pepper

Procedure

- Preheat oven to 350°F (175°C), sauté onion and garlic in the olive oil for about 3- 5 minutes, add mushroom thyme and finally spinach.

- Whisk eggs in a bowl, and add sautéed vegetables, dill, pepper, and cheese. Stir in the sautéed mushroom-spinach mixture

- Pour the mixture into a greased baking dish and bake until the center of the frittata is firm. (about 20-25)

Turkey and Vegetable Stir-Fry

INGREDIENTS: **4 servings**

1 lb. boneless turkey breast, sliced (chicken can also do)

2 cups broccoli florets

1 cup sliced carrots

1 bell pepper, sliced

2 cloves garlic, minced

2 tablespoons low-sodium soy sauce

1 tablespoon olive oil

2 tablespoons honey

1 teaspoon cornstarch

2 tablespoons vinegar

1 teaspoon grated ginger (optional)

Procedure

- Stir together vinegar, cornstarch, honey, and soy sauce and set aside.

- Heat olive oil in a pan, add garlic and ginger, and vegetables, stir for a minute or until tender

- Set aside the vegetable and in the hot skillet stir fry the turkey until it is no longer pink. Make a space in the middle of the skillet Pour in the sauce in the middle of the skillet and cook until thickened.

- Pour in the vegetables and stir all ingredients together to coat, cook until heated through.

- Serve immediately over rice

Tuna and White Bean Salad

INGREDIENTS: **4 servings**

2 cans tuna, drained and flaked

2 cups cannellini beans (no salt added) drained

½ cup diced red onion

¼ cup chopped fresh parsley

2 tablespoon dill pickles cut into bite-size

2 tablespoons olive oil

2 tablespoons red wine vinegar

¼ teaspoon pepper

Procedure

- Mix beans, red onion, pickles, olive oil, vinegar, and pepper in a bowl, divide between the plates, and top with tuna and parsley.

Spinach feta stuffed chicken breast

INGREDIENTS   4 servings

4 boneless, skinless chicken breasts

2 cups fresh spinach, chopped

½ cup low-sodium chicken broth

½ cup crumbled feta cheese

2 tablespoons chopped dill

1 medium onion

2 cloves garlic, minced

1 tablespoon olive oil

Salt and pepper to taste

Toothpicks or kitchen twine for securing

procedure

- Preheat oven to 375 °f, in a large skillet sauté the onion and minced garlic until fragrant, add the chopped spinach and stir until wilted, add the chicken broth and cook for about 2 minutes, remove skillet from heat and allow to cool, once cooled stir in the feat chees, season with and pepper.

- Cut horizontally through the center of each chicken breast to form pockets, be careful not to cut all the way through.

- Spoon the spinach and feta mixture into the pockets of each chicken breast, dividing it evenly among them. Secure the openings with toothpicks or kitchen twine to keep the filling inside.

- Place the stuffed chicken in an oven-safe dish or foil, and bake in the preheated oven for about 25-30 minutes or the internal temperature runs 165°f. garnish with fresh dill and serve

Baked Cod with Herbs

INGREDIENTS: 4 servings

4 cod fillets

2 tablespoons chopped fresh parsley

1 tablespoon chopped fresh dill

2 tablespoons olive oil

½ ground rosemary

2 cloves garlic, minced

½ teaspoon black pepper

Salt to taste (optional)

Procedure

- Preheat oven to 350°f,
- Mix parsley, dill, olive oil, garlic, salt, rosemary, and pepper. Rub onto cod fillets and bake for 15-25 minutes.
- Serve with steamed vegetables or quinoa salad.

Turkey and Bean Chili

INGREDIENTS:

1 lb. ground lean turkey

2 cans of low-sodium kidney beans, drained

1 can dice tomatoes

1 onion, diced

2 cloves garlic, minced

2 tablespoons chili powder

1 tablespoon olive oil

1 teaspoon cumin

1 medium bell pepper

Salt and pepper to taste

Procedure

- Sauté onion, garlic, green pepper, and turkey until tender and turkey browned, Add beans, diced tomatoes, chili powder, cumin, salt, and pepper. Simmer for 20-25 minutes. Garnish with shredded cheese if desired.

Stuffed Bell Peppers

INGREDIENTS: **4 servings**

4 bell peppers, halved and seeds removed

1 cup cooked brown rice

1 cup black beans, drained and rinsed

1 cup diced tomatoes

1/2 cup diced onion

1/2 cup shredded low-fat cheese

2 cloves garlic, minced

2 tablespoons olive oil

1 teaspoon dried oregano

1 teaspoon cumin

Fresh dill or parsley for garnish

Salt and pepper to taste

Procedure

- Preheat oven to 375°F (190°C). Place bell pepper halves in a baking dish.

- In a pan, sauté onion, garlic, and dried oregano in olive oil until soft. Add cooked rice, black beans, diced tomatoes, cumin, salt, and pepper. Cook for a few minutes.

- Spoon the mixture into the bell pepper halves. Top with shredded cheese. Bake for 25-30 minutes.

Note: you can enjoy this recipe with grounded beef, ground turkey, or chicken if desired

Roasted Vegetable and Chicken Quinoa Bowl

INGREDIENTS:

2 cups cooked quinoa

1 lb. chicken breast, grilled and sliced

2 cups mixed roasted vegetables (bell peppers, zucchini, mushroom, broccoli, carrot, eggplant)

¼ cup crumbled feta cheese

½ tablespoon curry powder

2 tablespoons chopped fresh parsley

2 tablespoons balsamic glaze

Salt and pepper to taste

Olive oil

Chicken stock

Procedure

- Preheat oven to 400°f, in a large bowel mix together the vegetables with salt, pepper, and garlic powder and bake until the vegetables are tender or have a nice brown color

- Meanwhile to cook quinoa, bring chicken stock to a boil and cook according to package instructions. In a skillet cook the chicken until browned and cooked.

- Divide cooked quinoa into bowls.

- Top with grilled chicken slices, roasted vegetables, crumbled feta cheese, and parsley.

- Drizzle with balsamic glaze and season with salt and pepper.

Greek Lemon Chicken Soup (Avgolemono)

INGREDIENTS: **4-6 servings**

6 cups low-sodium chicken broth

1 lb. boneless, skinless chicken breast

½ cup uncooked white rice

2 eggs

1 medium carrot

2 garlic cloves minced

Juice of 2 lemons

2 bay leaves

Zest of 1 lemon

½ onion

I tablespoon cornstarch (optional)

Salt and pepper to taste

Chopped fresh dill for garnish (optional)

Note: you can use 3 cups of water and three cups of stock.

Procedure

- In a pot, bring chicken broth to a boil. Add chicken breast, onion, bay leaf, garlic, carrot and rice. Simmer for 20-25 minutes until chicken is cooked and rice is tender.

- Remove the chicken, shred it, and return to the pot.

- In a bowl or blender whisk together eggs, lemon juice, cornstarch if using, and lemon zest. Slowly add a ladle of hot broth to the egg mixture, whisking constantly.

- Pour the egg-lemon mixture back into the pot while stirring constantly. Cook for a few more minutes without boiling. Season with salt and pepper and garnish with fresh dill on each plate.

CHAPTER 4: DINNER RECIPES

Shrimp and Asparagus Stir-Fry

INGREDIENTS: 4 servings

1 lb. shrimp, peeled and deveined

1 bunch asparagus, trimmed and cut into pieces

2 cloves garlic, minced

2 tablespoons low-sodium soy sauce

1 tablespoon sesame oil

1 tablespoon cornstarch

1 onion

2 tablespoons vegetable oil

procedure

- In a bowl, mix soy sauce, sesame oil, and cornstarch. Add shrimp and toss to coat.

- Heat vegetable oil in a pan over high heat. Add minced garlic, onions and stir-fry for 30 seconds.

- Add shrimp and marinade to the pan. Stir-fry for 2-3 minutes for the shrimps to turn pink

- Add asparagus and continue stir-frying for an additional 2-3 minutes until asparagus is tender.

Chicken and Broccoli Alfredo

INGREDIENTS: **4-5 servings**

8 oz whole wheat fettuccine pasta

2 boneless, skinless chicken breasts, cut into strips

2 cups broccoli florets

2 cloves garlic, minced

1 cup low-sodium chicken broth or lemon juice

1 cup low-fat milk or half-and-half creamer

¼ cup grated Parmesan cheese

1 teaspoon ground peppercorn

2 tablespoons olive oil

Red bell pepper for garnish (optional)

pepper to taste

Procedure

- Cook pasta according to package instructions without salt add broccoli in the last minutes and drain.

- Heat olive oil in a pan over medium heat, add chicken strips and minced garlic, cook until browned.

- Pour in chicken broth, and milk, and bring to a boil Stir in cooked pasta, peppercorn, garlic powder, and grated Parmesan cheese. Cook for a few more minutes until the sauce thickens, sprinkle with pepper and bell pepper.

Baked Vegetable Ratatouille Pasta

INGREDIENTS: **4 servings**

8 oz whole grain pasta

1 eggplant, diced

2 zucchinis, diced

1 bell pepper, diced

2 cups marinara sauce

1 medium onion diced

2 garlic cloves minced

3-4 tomatoes (optional)

1/2 cup grated Parmesan cheese

2 tablespoons olive oil

1 tablespoon balsamic vinegar (optional)

Salt and pepper to taste

Fresh dill or parsley for garnishing

Procedure

- Preheat oven to 375°F (190°C), Cook pasta according to package instructions, and drain.

- In a baking dish, combine diced eggplant, zucchini, bell pepper, marinara sauce, olive oil, onion, tomatoes, minced garlic, salt, and pepper. Bake for 25-30 minutes or until vegetables are tender.

- Mix the baked vegetables with cooked pasta, sprinkle grated Parmesan cheese and fresh parsley if using, and serve.

Veggie Lentil Burgers

INGREDIENTS: **4 servings**

1 cup cooked lentils

1 cup chopped mixed vegetables (bell peppers, carrots, onions)

1/2 cup breadcrumbs

1 egg

2 tablespoons olive oil

1 teaspoon paprika

½ teaspoon dried oregano

2 tablespoons walnuts chopped (optional)

¼ teaspoon garlic powder

Salt and pepper to taste

procedure

- In a bowl, mash cooked lentils. Add chopped vegetables, breadcrumbs, egg, garlic, walnuts, paprika, salt, and pepper. Mix well.

- Form the mixture into burger patties, Heat olive oil in a skillet over medium heat. Cook the patties until each side turns golden brown and cooked.

- Serve in buns or lettuce wraps with your favorite toppings adhering to renal-friendly ingredients.

Turkey and Spinach Stuffed Mushrooms

INGREDIENTS: **4-6 servings**

12 large button mushrooms, stems removed

½ lb. ground turkey

1 cup chopped spinach

¼ cup grated Parmesan cheese

2 cloves garlic, minced

1 tablespoon olive oil

1 medium onion

2 tablespoons bell pepper

¼ teaspoon paprika

Salt and pepper to taste

Procedure

- Preheat oven to 375°F (190°C). Heat olive oil in a skillet over medium heat and add minced garlic and onions, sauté for about a minute. Add ground turkey and cook until browned. Stir in chopped spinach, salt, pepper, and any other spice if using. Cook until spinach wilts.

- Fill mushroom caps with the turkey-spinach mixture and place them on a baking sheet.

- Sprinkle grated Parmesan cheese over the stuffed mushrooms and bake for about 15-20 minutes or until mushrooms are soft and tender.

Mediterranean Chickpea Salad

INGREDIENTS:

2 cans chickpeas, drained and rinsed

1 cucumber, diced

1 cup cherry tomatoes, halved

½ cup diced red onion

¼ cup chopped fresh parsley

¼ cup chopped fresh mint

2 tablespoons olive oil

2 tablespoons red wine vinegar

2-ounce feta cheese (optional)

2 tablespoons lemon juice

pepper to taste

Procedure

- In a large bowl, combine chickpeas, diced cucumber, cherry tomatoes, red onion, parsley, and mint. Chop cheese into bite size and add to bowl if using

- sprinkle olive oil, lemon, and red wine vinegar over the salad. Toss thoroughly to combine.

- Serve with grilled chicken and enjoy.

Lemon Herb Baked Pork Chops

Ingredients: 4 servings

4 pork chops

2 tablespoons olive oil

3 cloves garlic, minced

½ teaspoon paprika

1 lemon (Zest and juice)

1 tablespoon chopped fresh rosemary or ½ teaspoon dried

½ teaspoon thyme

½ teaspoon ground oregano

Salt and pepper to taste

Procedure

- Preheat oven to 375°F (190°C). Mix olive oil, minced garlic, lemon zest, lemon juice, chopped rosemary, thyme, paprika, salt, and pepper in a bowl.

- Rub and mix the mixture with the pork and allow it to rest for some time to marinate. the pork chops with this mixture allow

- Place pork chops in a baking dish and bake for 25-30 minutes or until cooked through.

- Serve with roasted vegetables and enjoy.

Sweet Potato and Black Bean Quesadillas

INGREDIENTS: 4 servings

2 medium sweet potatoes, peeled and diced

1 can low-sodium black beans, drained and rinsed

1 teaspoon ground cumin

1 teaspoon chili powder

½ teaspoon paprika

½ onion

1 medium bell pepper

4 whole wheat tortillas

1 cup shredded low-fat cheese

Olive oil for cooking

Procedure

- Boil, steam or roast diced sweet potatoes until tender. Mash them in a bowl and mix in black beans, cumin, paprika, and chili powder.

- In a skillet, sauté onion, garlic if using, and bell pepper until translucent. Mix it in the potato bowl.

- Spread the sweet potato and black bean mixture on one half of each tortilla, sprinkle with shredded cheese, then fold in half.

- Heat olive oil in a skillet over medium heat. Cook each quesadilla for 2-3 minutes on each side until golden and crispy.

Ratatouille

INGREDIENTS: **4-7 servings**

1 eggplant, diced

2 zucchinis, diced

2 carrots diced

1 red bell pepper, diced

1 green bell pepper diced

2 tomatoes, diced

1 large onion, diced

3 cloves garlic, minced

2 tablespoons olive oil

1 tablespoon of fresh rosemary

1 tablespoon zest (optional)

1 tablespoon fresh basil

1 teaspoon dried thyme

8 tablespoons grated parmesan cheese (optional)

Ground black pepper to taste

Procedure

- Heat olive oil in a skillet over medium heat and add diced onion and garlic, cook until softened. Add diced eggplant, zucchini, bell peppers, zest if using, basil, rosemary, thyme, and pepper. Cook for 10-15 minutes or until tender stirring occasionally.

- Add the tomatoes and cheese if using and mix well, simmering covered until vegetables are ready. Serve hot as a side dish or add pasta, you can also add cooked ground turkey, chicken, or beef to make it whole.

Shrimp and Veggie Skillet

INGREDIENTS:

1 lb. shrimp, peeled and deveined

2 cups mixed vegetables (zucchini, bell peppers, broccoli, squash)

2 tablespoons olive oil

2 cloves garlic, minced

½ tablespoon cumin

½ onion diced

Fresh parsley for garnishing

1 teaspoon smoked paprika

pepper to taste

Procedure

- Mix the shrimp with pepper, paprika, and cumin, and Heat olive oil in a skillet on medium heat, add minced garlic with onion and cook for 1 minute.

- Add shrimp and cook until it's about 2 minutes, add the vegetables and add the remaining smoked paprika, cumin, and pepper. Stir-fry until shrimp is pink and vegetables are tender and sprinkle fresh parsley.

- Serve with cauliflower rice or brown rice if desired.

Veggie Packed Turkey Meatballs

INGREDIENTS: **4 servings**

1 lb. ground turkey

½ cup grated zucchini

½ cup grated carrot

¼ cup chopped spinach

¼ cup breadcrumbs

2 garlic cloves minced

½ onion minced

1 egg

2 tablespoons chopped fresh parsley

pepper to taste

Procedure

- Preheat oven to 400°F and Line a baking sheet with parchment paper.

- In a bowl, combine ground turkey, grated zucchini, grated carrot, chopped spinach, breadcrumbs, egg, onion, garlic, parsley, salt, and pepper. Mix well.

- Form mixture into meatballs and place them on the prepared baking sheet.

- Bake for about 20-25 minutes or until meatballs are done and cooked through. Serve with vegetables or salad

Veggie Quinoa Bowl

INGREDIENTS: **2-4 servings**

2 cups cooked quinoa

1 cup cooked black beans

1 cup cooked corn kernels

1 avocado, sliced

1 cup cherry tomatoes, halved

2 tablespoons sesame seed roasted

1/4 cup chopped cilantro

Lime wedges for serving

Procedure

- Divide cooked quinoa into bowls. Top with black beans, corn kernels, sesame seeds, avocado slices, cherry tomatoes, and chopped cilantro.
- Serve with lime wedges for squeezing over the bowl.

Beef Stir-Fry with Broccoli and Mushrooms

INGREDIENTS: **4 servings**

1 lb. beef sirloin, thinly sliced

2 cups broccoli florets

1 cup sliced mushrooms

½ red bell pepper sliced

2 tablespoons low-sodium soy sauce

1 tomatoes diced (optional)

1 tablespoon cornstarch

2 cloves garlic, minced

½ cup low-sodium chicken broth

2 tablespoons vegetable (peanut)

Procedure

- Heat oil in a wok or skillet and sauté garlic until fragrant, add the vegetables and stir until tender, remove the vegetables and set aside.
- In the same skillet, stir fry the chicken until cooked, and in a bowl mix soy sauce, cornstarch, and stock.
- Add the sauce, and tomatoes to the skillet and stir, add vegetables, and heat until the sauce is thick.
- Serve on rice.

Blackened Tilapia with Mango Salsa

INGREDIENTS: **4 servings**

4 tilapia fillets

2 teaspoons paprika

1 teaspoon dried thyme

1 teaspoon onion powder

1 teaspoon garlic powder

1/2 teaspoon cayenne pepper

½ teaspoon black pepper

1/2 teaspoon salt

1 tablespoon fresh minced parsley

2 tablespoons olive oil

For Mango Salsa:

1 ripe mango, diced

½ red onion, finely chopped

¼ cup chopped fresh cilantro

Juice of 1 lime

Salt and pepper to taste

Procedure

- In a small bowl, mix paprika, thyme, onion powder, garlic powder, cayenne pepper, black pepper, parsley, lemon juice and salt. Rub this spice mixture onto both sides of the tilapia fillets and refrigerate in a resealable bag to marinate for about an hour.
- Heat olive oil in a skillet. Cook the tilapia for 3-4 minutes on each side until the fish is blackened and cooked through.
- For the mango salsa, combine diced mango, chopped red onion, cilantro, lime juice, and salt in a bowl. Mix well and Serve the blackened tilapia topped with mango salsa.

Turkey and Vegetable Soup with Barley

INGREDIENTS: **6-8 servings**

1 lb. ground turkey

1 cup chopped carrots

1 cup chopped celery

1 onion, diced

3 cloves garlic, minced

1 cup pearl barley

8 cups low-sodium chicken broth

1 teaspoon dried oregano

1 teaspoon dried thyme

Olive oil

Salt and pepper to taste

Procedure

- In a large pot, brown ground turkey over medium heat until cooked. Drain any excess fat.
- Add chopped carrots, celery, diced onion, and minced garlic. Cook for a few minutes until vegetables soften.
- Stir in pearl barley, chicken broth, dried thyme, salt, and pepper. Bring to a boil, then reduce heat and simmer for 30-40 minutes or until barley is tender.

Spinach and Mushroom Quiche

INGREDIENTS: 6 servings

1 refrigerated pie crust

6 eggs

1 cup chopped spinach

1 cup sliced mushrooms

1 cup onion sliced

½ cup low-fat milk

½ cup half and half ca reamer

1 cup shredded low-fat cheese

½ teaspoon dried thyme

2 garlic minced

1 tablespoon Dijon mustard

Salt and pepper to taste

Procedure

- Preheat oven to 375°F (190°C). Press the pie crust into a pie dish and flute the edges.
- In a skillet, sauté sliced mushrooms until brown and add onion, garlic, and spinach until tender.
- In a bowl, whisk together eggs, milk, dried thyme, mustard, creamer, salt, and pepper, mix in the vegetables and combine.

- Spread the spinach and mushrooms mixture in the pie crust. Pour the egg mixture over the filling.
- Bake for 30 to 35 minutes or until the quiche is set and the top is golden brown.

Veggie Lentil Curry

INGREDIENTS: 6 servings

1 cup dried red lentils

1 onion, diced

2 cloves garlic, minced

1 tablespoon curry powder

1 teaspoon ground cumin

1 teaspoon ground coriander

1 can (14 ounces) diced tomatoes

1 can (14 ounces) coconut milk

2 cups chopped mixed vegetables (cauliflower, bell peppers, carrots)

2 tablespoons olive oil

Salt and pepper to taste

Vegetable stock

procedure

- Rinse red lentils under cold water and drain.

- Heat olive oil in a pot over medium heat. Add diced onion and minced garlic, and cook until softened.
- Add in curry powder, ground cumin, and ground coriander. Cook for 1-2 minutes until fragrant.
- Add diced tomatoes, coconut milk, chopped mixed vegetables, and rinsed lentils. Bring to a simmer and cook for 20-25 minutes until vegetables and lentils are tender.
- Season with salt and pepper. Serve with rice or naan bread.

Spaghetti Squash with Tomato Sauce

INGREDIENTS: 4 servings

1 medium spaghetti squash

2 cups low-sodium tomato sauce

1 teaspoon dried basil

1 medium shallot diced

1 teaspoon dried oregano

2 cloves garlic, minced

2 tablespoons olive oil

 pepper to taste

Procedure

- Preheat oven to 400°F. Cut spaghetti squash in half lengthwise, scoop out seeds, and place face down on a baking sheet. Bake for 30-40 minutes.

- Heat olive oil in a pan, add garlic and shallot, and sauté until fragrant. Pour in tomato sauce, basil, oregano, and pepper. Simmer for 10-15 minutes.
- Scrape cooked spaghetti squash with a fork to create "noodles". Serve topped with tomato sauce. Serve As a pasta alternative with a side of steamed vegetables.

Vegetarian Lentil Tacos

INGREDIENTS: **4 servings**

1 cup cooked lentils

1 cup diced tomatoes

1/2 cup diced onion

1/2 cup chopped cilantro

2 tablespoons taco seasoning

1 tablespoon olive oil

8 whole grain taco shells

Optional toppings: shredded lettuce, diced avocado, Greek yogurt

Procedure

- Heat olive oil in a pan, and sauté onion until translucent. Add lentils, tomatoes, vegetables,

taco seasoning, and cilantro. Cook for 5-7 minutes.
- Fill taco shells with lentil mixture and desired toppings.

Greek Yogurt Chicken Salad

INGREDIENTS: **4 servings**

2 cups cooked shredded chicken

1/2 cup diced celery

1/2 cup halved grapes

1/4 cup chopped walnuts (optional)

1/2 cup Greek yogurt

2 tablespoons lemon juice

Salt and pepper to taste

Procedure

- Mix chicken, celery, grapes, and walnuts in a bowl.
- Stir in Greek yogurt, lemon juice, salt, and pepper.
- Serve As a sandwich filling or over lettuce leaves.

Mediterranean Style Baked Chicken

INGREDIENTS:

4 bone-in, skinless chicken thighs

1 tablespoon olive oil

2 cloves garlic, minced

1 teaspoon dried oregano

½ teaspoon paprika

¼ cup diced tomatoes

Salt and pepper to taste

Procedure

- Preheat oven to 375°F (190°C).
- Rub chicken thighs with olive oil, minced garlic, oregano, paprika, salt, and pepper.
- Place chicken in a baking dish, and and top with diced tomatoes.
- Bake for 35-40 minutes or until chicken is fully cooked.

CHAPTER 5: DESSERT RECIPE

Lemon Yogurt cake

INGREDIENTS: **8–10 slices**

1½ cups of flour for all purposes

½ cup almond flour

1 tsp baking powder

½ tsp baking soda

A pinch of salt

1 cup of Greek yogurt, plain

¾ cup of sugar, granulated

3 big eggs

 lemon's zest of 1 lemon

¼ cup of newly squeezed lemon juice

½ teaspoon vanilla extract

¼ cup vegetable oil

procedure

- Set oven temperature to 175°C/350°F. Apply grease to a loaf pan.
- Mix the flour, baking soda, baking powder, and salt in a bowl.
- Combine yogurt, sugar, eggs, lemon zest, lemon juice, vanilla extract, and vegetable oil in a

separate bowl and whisk until thoroughly blended.

- Gradually add the dry ingredients to the wet ones, mixing just until combined. After the loaf pan is ready, pour the batter into it.
- A toothpick inserted into the center should come out clean after 45 to 50 minutes of baking.
- After letting the cake set in the pan for ten minutes, turn it out onto a wire rack to finish cooling.
- Garnish slices with fresh berries or a dollop of low-phosphorus whipped topping.

Carrot Cake Muffins

INGREDIENTS: **12 muffins**

1 ½ cups grated carrots

½ cup whole wheat flour

½ cup all-purpose flour

½ cup rolled oats

1 teaspoon baking powder

½ teaspoon baking soda

1 teaspoon ground cinnamon

¼ teaspoon ground nutmeg

¼ teaspoon salt

½ cup unsweetened applesauce

¼ cup honey, maple syrup

¼ cup vegetable oil

2 large eggs

1 teaspoon vanilla extract

½ cup chopped walnuts (optional)

Procedure

- Set oven temperature to 175°C/350°F. Use paper liners to line a muffin tray.
- flour, oats, baking soda, baking powder, nutmeg, cinnamon, and salt should all be combined in a basin.
- Combine applesauce, eggs, vegetable oil, honey or maple syrup, and vanilla extract in a separate bowl.
- Mix the dry and wet components until they are well blended. stir in grated carrot, if using, fold in chopped walnuts, and distribute the batter among the muffin tins.
- When a toothpick put into the center comes out clean, bake for 18 to 20 minutes.

Baked cinnamon apples

INGREDIENTS: **8 half apples**

4 apples, cored and cut in half (preferably Granny Smith or Honeycrisp).

2 tsp melted unsalted butter

2 tsp honey or maple syrup

1 tsp finely ground cinnamon

chopped nuts (almond), optional for garnishing

procedure

- Turn the oven on to 375°F, or 190°C. Apple halves should be put in a baking dish.
- Combine cinnamon, honey (or maple syrup), and melted butter in a small bowl. Over the apple halves, pour the butter mixture.
- Bake the apples for 25 to 30 minutes, or until they are soft. If desired, top the baked apples with chopped nuts.

Angel Food Cake with Fresh Berries

INGREDIENTS: **10-12 servings**

1 ¼ cups egg whites (about 9 large eggs)

1 cup granulated sugar

1 cup cake flour

1 teaspoon cream of tartar

1 teaspoon vanilla extract

Fresh berries (strawberries, blueberries, raspberries) for topping

Procedure

- Preheat oven to 350°F (175°C). In a large mixing bowl, beat egg whites until frothy.

- Add cream of tartar and continue beating until soft peaks form. Gradually add powdered sugar while continuing to beat until stiff peaks form. Gently fold in cake flour and vanilla extract until well combined.
- Pour the batter into an ungreased angel food cake pan. Bake for 35-40 minutes or until the top is lightly golden and the cake springs back when touched. Invert the pan onto a cooling rack and let it cool completely before removing the cake. Top slices of angel food cake with fresh berries before serving.

Lemon Blueberry Cheesecake Bites

INGREDIENTS: **6-8 cheesecake bite**

1 cup low-fat cream cheese

1/4 cup Greek yogurt

Zest of 1 lemon

2 tablespoons fresh lemon juice

2-3 tablespoons honey or sugar substitute

1/2 teaspoon vanilla extract

Fresh blueberries for topping

Procedure

- In a mixing bowl, combine the low-fat cream cheese, Greek yogurt, lemon zest, lemon juice, honey (or sugar substitute), and vanilla extract.

Mix until smooth and well combined. Spoon the cheesecake mixture into small serving cups or molds. Refrigerate for at least 2-3 hours to allow the cheesecake bites to set.

Note: you can enjoy this recipe with graham cracker crumbs by firstly mixing it with butter, spread in a baking dish, and baking for about five minutes, then scoop the mixture on the crust and refrigerate.

Pumpkin Spice Muffins

INGREDIENTS: 10-12 muffins

1 cup all-purpose flour

¾ cup whole-wheat flour

1 teaspoon baking soda

½ teaspoon baking powder

½ teaspoon salt

1 teaspoon ground cinnamon

½ teaspoon ground nutmeg

½ teaspoon ground ginger

¼ teaspoon ground cloves

1 cup canned pumpkin puree

½ cup unsweetened applesauce

¼ cup vegetable oil

1 cup granulated sugar (or sugar substitute)

2 large eggs

1 teaspoon vanilla extract

Procedure

- Turn the oven on to 375°F, or 190°C. Use paper liners to line a muffin tray.
- Mix the flour, baking powder, baking soda, salt, cloves, nutmeg, and cinnamon in a basin.
- Pumpkin puree, applesauce, vegetable oil, sugar, eggs, and vanilla extract should all be thoroughly mixed in a separate basin.
- Mix the dry ingredients to the wet ones until incorporated thoroughly, Pour the mixture into the muffin tins.
- Bake for about 20-25 minutes or until toothpick or tester inserted inside out clean.

Banana Walnut Bread

INGREDIENTS: **1 loaf (8-10 slices)**

3 ripe bananas, mashed

1/3 cup unsweetened applesauce

¼ cup vegetable oil

½ cup granulated sugar (or sugar substitute)

1 teaspoon vanilla extract

1 cups all-purpose flour

½ cup oat flour

1 teaspoon baking soda

¼ teaspoon salt

½ cup chopped walnuts

procedure

- Preheat oven to 350°F (175°C). Grease a loaf pan. In a large bowl, mix mashed bananas, applesauce, vegetable oil, sugar, and vanilla extract.
- Mix the flour, baking soda, and salt in a separate bowl. Stirring until just blended, gradually add the dry ingredients to the wet components. Add the chopped walnuts and fold. pour the batter into the set loaf pan.
- Bake for 50 -60 minutes or until the tester comes out clean when inserted in the middle.
- Allow the banana walnut bread to cool in the pan for 10 minutes before transferring it to a wire rack to cool completely.

Mango Sorbet

INGREDIENTS: **3-4 servings**

4 ripe mangoes, peeled and diced

¼ cup honey or sugar substitute

2 tablespoons fresh lime or lemon juice

½ cup water

Procedure

- Pour the diced mangoes into a food processor or blender, Add honey (or sugar substitute) and lime or lemon juice.
- Blend until smooth. If the mixture is too thick, add water gradually while blending until desired consistency is reached.
- Transfer the mixture to a shallow dish and freeze for 3-4 hours, stirring every 30 minutes to break up ice crystals until it's firm but scoopable. Once properly frozen, scoop into serving bowls or cones.

Coconut Rice Pudding

INGREDIENTS: 4 servings

1 cup white rice (short or medium-grain)

4 cups coconut milk

¼ cup granulated sugar (or sugar substitute)

1 teaspoon vanilla extract

¼ cup shredded unsweetened coconut (optional)

Ground cinnamon for garnish (optional)

Procedure

- Till the water runs clear, rinse the rice under cold water. Place the rice and coconut milk in a saucepan. Over medium heat, bring it to a boil, and then turn down the heat.

- Cover and simmer for 20 to 25 minutes, stirring from time to time, or until the rice is soft and the mixture has thickened.
- Add the sugar, crushed coconut (if using), and vanilla essence. Cook the pudding for a further five to ten minutes, or until the consistency you like is reached. Turn off the heat and let it cool. Serve warm or cold, topped, if preferred, with ground cinnamon.

Almond Flour Chocolate Cake

INGREDIENTS: **8-10 servings**

2 cups almond flour

½ cup unsweetened cocoa powder

1 teaspoon baking soda

¼ teaspoon salt

½ cup unsweetened applesauce

¼ cup vegetable oil

¾ cup granulated sugar (or sugar substitute)

4 large eggs

1 teaspoon vanilla extract

Procedure

- Preheat oven to 350°F (175°C). Grease a cake pan. In a bowl, whisk together almond flour, cocoa powder, baking soda, and salt.

- In another bowl, mix applesauce, vegetable oil, sugar, eggs, and vanilla extract until well combined. Gradually add the dry ingredients to the wet ingredients, stirring until thoroughly combined.
- Transfer the mixture into the ready-made cake pan. bake for 30 to 35 minutes or when a toothpick put into the center comes out clean, after letting the cake set in the pan for 10 minutes, turn it out onto a wire rack to finish cooling.

Chocolate Banana Bread

INGREDIENTS: **1 loaf (8-10 slices)**

3 ripe bananas, mashed

1/ cup unsweetened applesauce

¼ cup vegetable oil

2/3 cup granulated sugar

1 teaspoon vanilla extract

1 ¾ cups all-purpose flour

¼ cup unsweetened cocoa powder

1 teaspoon baking soda

½ teaspoon salt

½ cup semi-sweet chocolate chips

Procedure

- Preheat oven to 350°F (175°C). Grease a loaf pan. In a large mixing bowl, combine mashed bananas, applesauce, vegetable oil, sugar, and vanilla extract.
- In another bowl, whisk together flour, cocoa powder, baking soda, and salt. Add the dry ingredients to the wet components little by little and stir until just blended. Add the chocolate chips and fold.
- Fill the prepared loaf pan with the batter. Bake for about 50-60 minutes or until a toothpick inserted in the center comes out clean. After 10 minutes of cooling in the pan, move the bread to a wire rack to finish cooling.

Vanilla Panna Cotta with Raspberry Sauce

INGREDIENTS: **4 servings**

2 cups low-fat milk

¼ cup granulated sugar (or sugar substitute)

1 teaspoon vanilla extract

2 teaspoons unflavored gelatin

2 tablespoons cold water

1 cup fresh or frozen raspberries

2 tablespoons water

1-2 tablespoons honey or sugar (optional)

Plain yogurt or whipped cream (optional)

Procedure

- In a saucepan, heat the milk and sugar over medium heat until it's warm but not boiling. Add in the vanilla extract and remove from heat.
- In a small bowl, sprinkle gelatin over cold water and let it sit for a few minutes to soften. Add the softened gelatin to the warm milk mixture and whisk until completely dissolved.
- Pour the mixture into individual serving cups or ramekins. Refrigerate for at least 2-4 hours or until set.
- For the raspberry sauce, in a small saucepan, combine raspberries, water, and honey or sugar (if using). Simmer over medium heat until the raspberries soften and the sauce starts to get somewhat thicker. Take off from heat and filter using a fine-mesh strainer to eliminate the seeds. After the panna cotta sets, drizzle the raspberry sauce over it.

Avocado Chocolate Mousse

INGREDIENTS: **4 servings**

2 ripe avocados, peeled and pitted

¼ cup unsweetened cocoa powder

¼ cup honey or sugar substitute

1 teaspoon vanilla extract

Pinch of salt

Fresh berries for garnish (optional)

Procedure

- In a food processor or blender, combine the avocados, cocoa powder, honey (or sugar substitute), vanilla extract, and salt. Blend until smooth and creamy, scraping down the sides as needed to ensure everything is mixed well.
- Divide the chocolate mousse into serving cups or bowls. Refrigerate for at least 30 minutes to chill and serve. Before serving, garnish with fresh berries if desired.

Orange Almond Cake

INGREDIENTS: 8-10 servings

1 ½ cups almond flour

½ cup granulated sugar (or sugar substitute)

Zest of 1 orange

½ teaspoon baking powder

¼ teaspoon salt

3 large eggs

¼ cup vegetable oil

2 tablespoons fresh orange juice

1 teaspoon vanilla extract

Procedure

- Preheat oven to 350°F (175°C). Grease a cake pan. In a bowl, whisk together almond flour, sugar, orange zest, baking powder, and salt.
- In another bowl, beat eggs, vegetable oil, orange juice, and vanilla extract until well combined. Add the dry ingredients to the wet components little by little and stir until just blended.
- Fill the prepared cake pan with the batter. Bake for about 30-35 minutes or until a toothpick inserted in the middle comes out clear.

Gingerbread Cookies

INGREDIENTS: **24 cookies**

2 cups all-purpose flour

1 teaspoon baking soda

1 teaspoon ground ginger

1 teaspoon ground cinnamon

¼ teaspoon ground cloves

½ cup unsalted butter, softened

½ cup brown sugar or granulated sugar

¼ cup molasse or honey

2 egg whites

Low-phosphorus icing (optional)

Procedure

- Combine the flour, baking soda, cloves, ginger, cinnamon, and salt in a bowl. Creamy butter and brown sugar should be combined in a separate basin.
- Beat the egg and molasses into the butter mixture thoroughly. Mixing until mixed, gradually add the dry ingredients to the wet ones.
- Split the dough in half, press the dough into discs, cover with plastic wrap, and chill for a minimum of two hours. Set oven temperature to 175°C/350°F. Use parchment paper to line baking sheets.
- Roll out the dough to a thickness of approximately 1/4 inch on a surface dusted with flour. Cut into the appropriate shapes using cookie cutters.
- Lay out cookies on baking sheets that have been prepped, and bake for 8 to 10 minutes, or until edges are hard. If you would like to decorate the cookies with low-phosphorus icing, wait until they are cool.

Date and Walnut Bars

INGREDIENTS: **8-10 bars**

1 cup pitted dates, chopped

¼ cup water

1 teaspoon vanilla extract

1 cup oat flour (finely ground oats)

½ teaspoon baking soda

¼ teaspoon salt

½ cup chopped walnuts

Procedure

- Set oven temperature to 175°C/350°F. A baking pan can be lined with parchment paper or greased. Add the water and chopped dates to a saucepan. Cook, stirring periodically, over medium heat until dates soften and take on the consistency of paste.
- Take it off the stove, mix in the vanilla essence, and allow it to cool a little. Combine the oat flour, baking soda, salt, and chopped walnuts in another basin.
- Mix the dry ingredients with the date mixture until a dough forms. Using the prepared baking pan, press the dough evenly.
- Bake until the edges are golden brown, 15 to 18 minutes. Let it cool down in the pan entirely before slicing into bars.

Black Forest Chia Seed Pudding

INGREDIENTS: **2 servings**

¼ cup chia seeds

1 cup unsweetened almond milk (or any preferred milk)

1 tablespoon cocoa powder

1-2 tablespoons honey or sugar substitute

1/4 teaspoon almond extract (optional)

Low-phosphorus whipped topping (optional)

Fresh cherries or canned cherries in juice (for topping)

Procedure

- In a bowl, mix chia seeds, almond milk, cocoa powder, honey (or sugar substitute), and almond extract (if using). Stir well to combine all ingredients.
- Cover the bowl and refrigerate for at least 2 hours or overnight to allow the chia seeds to gel and thicken.
- Once the pudding is set, layer it in serving cups or bowls, alternating with layers of low-phosphorus whipped topping and fresh or canned cherries. Garnish with additional cherries on top before serving.

Pineapple Upside-Down Cake

INGREDIENTS: 8-10 servings

1 can pineapple slices in juice, drained or 1 whole pineapple peeled, cored, and cut in ring form.

¼ cup unsalted butter, melted (optional)

½ cup brown sugar (or sugar substitute)

Maraschino cherries, drained

1 ½ cups all-purpose flour

1 teaspoon baking powder

¼ teaspoon salt

½ cup unsweetened applesauce or milk

½ cup granulated sugar (or sugar substitute)

2 large eggs

1 teaspoon vanilla extract

procedure

- Set oven temperature to 175°C/350°F. Oil a circular cake pan. Place the pineapple slices in the cake pan's bottom. Put a cherry in the middle of every slice of pineapple.
- Dust the pineapple slices and cherries with brown sugar. Pour melted butter over the top.
- Mix the flour, baking powder, and salt in a bowl. Combine applesauce, eggs, granulated sugar, and vanilla extract in a separate basin and whisk thoroughly.
- Mixing until mixed thoroughly, gradually add the dry ingredients to the wet ones. Over the pineapple slices in the pan, pour the batter.
- Bake for about 30-35 minutes or until the cake is set, let it cool for some minutes before turning it in the pan.

Honey Yogurt Parfait

INGREDIENTS: 2 servings

2 cups low-fat Greek yogurt

¼ cup honey

1 cup mixed fresh berries (such as strawberries, blueberries, raspberries)

¼ cup low phosphorus granola

Procedure

- In a bowl, mix Greek yogurt and honey until well combined. In serving glasses or bowls, layer the honey yogurt mixture, fresh berries, and granola. Repeat the layers as desired, ending with a sprinkle of granola on top.

Lemon Ricotta Cookies

INGREDIENTS: **24 cookies**

2 cups all-purpose flour

½ teaspoon baking powder

½ teaspoon baking soda

¼ teaspoon salt

½ cup unsalted butter, softened

1 cup granulated sugar (or sugar substitute)

1 cup ricotta cheese

1 large egg

2 tablespoons fresh lemon juice

Zest of 1 lemon

Powdered sugar for dusting (optional)

procedure

- Set oven temperature to 175°C/350°F. Use parchment paper to line baking sheets. Mix the flour, baking soda, baking powder, and salt in a bowl.
- Beat sugar and butter together in a separate dish until frothy and light. Stir in the egg, lemon zest, juice, and ricotta cheese. Blend until thoroughly blended. Mixing until mixed thoroughly, add the dry ingredients to the wet ones.
- Drop dough onto the prepared baking sheets by spoonful. Bake for 12 to 15 minutes, or until cookies are slightly brown around the edges and firm.
- After a few minutes, let the cookies cool on the baking sheets before moving them to a wire rack to finish cooling. If desired, dust with powdered sugar.

Raspberry Chia Seed Jam

INGREDIENTS: 1 jar

2 cups fresh raspberries

2 tablespoons honey or sugar substitute

2 tablespoons chia seeds

1 tablespoon fresh lemon juice

Procedure

- In a saucepan, cook raspberries and honey (or sugar substitute) over medium heat, stirring regularly, until the raspberries break down and turn syrupy.
- Mash the raspberries with a fork or potato masher.
- Stir in the chia seeds and lemon juice, then decrease the heat to low.
- Simmer for about 10-15 minutes, stirring often, until the sauce has thickened.
- Remove from heat and allow to cool. The jam will thicken as it cools.
- Place the jam in a jar or airtight container and chill. It will keep for around a week or can be frozen.

This recipe can be enjoyed as toppings for toast, desserts, or yogurts.

CHAPTER 6: SNACKS AND DRINKS

Greek Yogurt Parfait

INGREDIENTS:

1 cup low-fat Greek yogurt

1/2 cup fresh berries

2 tablespoons chopped nuts (almonds, walnuts)

Procedure

- Layer yogurt, berries, and nuts in a glass. Repeat layering and top with lemon zest and whipped cream if desired.

Cucumber Avocado Rolls

INGREDIENTS:

1 cucumber

1 avocado

1 teaspoon lemon juice

1 tablespoon diced bell pepper

¼ teaspoon paprika

Procedure

- Slice cucumber lengthwise into strips.
- Spread avocado mixed with lemon juice and pepper if desired on each strip, sprinkle with

diced bell pepper, and roll up, secure with a toothpick if desired, and sprinkle with paprika.

Roasted Chickpeas

INGREDIENTS:

1 can of 15-ounce chickpeas, drained and rinsed

1 tablespoon olive oil

1 teaspoon paprika

½ teaspoon garlic powder

½ teaspoon black pepper (optional

procedure

- Preheat oven to 400°F (200°C). Toss chickpeas with olive oil and spices, then spread on a baking sheet. Roast for 25-30 minutes until crispy.

Veggie Sticks with Hummus

INGREDIENTS:

2 carrots, cut into sticks

2 celery stalks, cut into sticks

½ cup hummus

procedure

- Arrange veggie sticks on a plate with a side of hummus.

Note: you can make a low-sodium homemade hummus with chickpea, lemon juice, tahini, garlic, olive oil, and blend

Cottage Cheese with Pineapple

INGREDIENTS:

½ cup low-fat cottage cheese

½ cup diced fresh or canned in-juice pineapple

Procedure

- Mix cottage cheese and diced pineapple, sprinkle chia seed on top if needed.

Berry Smoothie

INGREDIENTS:

½ cup mixed berries (strawberries, blueberries, raspberries)

1/2 cup unsweetened almond milk

½ cup low-fat yogurt

Maple syrup (optional)

Procedure

- Blend all ingredients until smooth.

Cucumber Mint Water

INGREDIENTS:

½ cucumber, sliced

a few sprigs of fresh mint

½ lemon sliced

4 cups water

Procedure

- Combine cucumber and mint in a pitcher of water and let it infuse in the fridge for a few hours.

Iced Chamomile Tea

INGREDIENTS:

2 chamomile tea bags

2 teaspoons honey

1 teaspoon fresh grated ginger

Lemon slices

1 teaspoon cumin (optional)

4 cups water

Ice cubes

Procedure

- Steep tea bags, ginger, lemon, and cumin in hot boiling water for about 15 minutes stirring, then sieve and let it cool. Serve over ice.

Pineapple Ginger Mocktail

INGREDIENTS:

1 cup pineapple juice

1 teaspoon grated ginger

1 teaspoon maple syrup (optional)

Sparkling water (optional)

Procedure

- Mix pineapple juice and grated ginger. Add sparkling water if desired and serve chilled.

Watermelon Slush

INGREDIENTS:

2 cups diced watermelon

Juice of 1 lime

Ice cubes

Procedure

- Blend watermelon and lime juice with ice until slushy.

Baked Sweet Potato Fries

INGREDIENTS:

2 sweet potatoes, cut into fries

1 tablespoon olive oil

½ teaspoon paprika

Procedure

- Preheat oven to 425°F (220°C). Toss sweet potato fries with olive oil and paprika, then spread on a baking sheet. Bake for 25-30 minutes until crispy.

Tuna Cucumber Bites

INGREDIENTS:

1 can (5 ounces) tuna, drained

1 cucumber, sliced (seedless)

2 tablespoons Greek yogurt

1 tablespoon chopped dill

½ onion diced (optional)

Ground pepper to taste

Procedure

- Mix tuna, Greek yogurt, onion, pepper, and dill. Place a spoonful of the tuna mixture on each cucumber slice.

Apple Cinnamon Oat Bars

INGREDIENTS:

2 cups rolled oats

1 cup unsweetened applesauce

1 teaspoon vanilla extract

1 apple peeled and grated

¼ teaspoon baking soda

2 tablespoons unsalted butter

2 tablespoons honey

1 teaspoon cinnamon

Procedure

- Preheat oven to 350°F (175°C). Mix all ingredients in a bowl. Press mixture into a lined baking pan and bake for 20–25 minutes.

Rice Cake with Almond Butter

INGREDIENTS:

1 rice cake

1 tablespoon almond butter

Procedure

- Spread almond butter over the rice cake.

Carrot Apple Juice

INGREDIENTS:

2 carrots

1 apple

Procedure

- Wash and chop carrots and apples into chunks. Juice the carrots and apples together. Dilute with water if desired. Serve chilled or over ice.

Lemon-Basil Infused Water

INGREDIENTS:

1 lemon, sliced

a handful of fresh basil leaves

4 cups water

Procedure

- Combine lemon slices and basil in a pitcher of water and refrigerate for a few hours.

Cranberry Spritzer

INGREDIENTS:

½ cup unsweetened cranberry juice

1 tablespoon lemon juice

Raspberry sherbet

Sparkling water

Fresh lime slices

Procedure

- Pour cranberry juice, lemon juice, and raspberry sherbet into a glass and top with sparkling water. Add lime slices for extra flavor if desired and serve chilled in a tall glass.

Herbal Iced Tea

INGREDIENTS:

2 herbal tea bags (such as hibiscus or mint)

4 cups water

Ice cubes

Procedure

- Steep herbal tea bags in hot water for 10 minutes, then let it cool and Serve over ice.

Trail Mix

INGREDIENTS: 6- 8 servings

1 cup unsalted almonds

1 cup unsalted cashews

1 cup unsalted pumpkin seeds

1 cup unsweetened dried cranberries

1 cup unsweetened dried apricots, chopped

½ cup unsweetened banana chips

½ teaspoon cinnamon (optional)

Procedure

- In a large mixing bowl, combine the almonds, cashews, pumpkin seeds, dried cranberries, chopped dried apricots, and banana chips.
- If desired, sprinkle cinnamon over the mix for added flavor. Toss the ingredients together until well combined.

Cherry Almond Smoothie

INGREDIENTS:

1 cup frozen cherries

1 tablespoon almond butter

½ cup plain Greek yogurt

½ cup almond milk

1 ripe banana

Spinach (optional: and will change the color)

Procedure

- Blend all ingredients until smooth and serve chilled.

BONUSES

TIPS TO HELP YOU STICK TO YOUR RENAL DIET

Sticking to a renal diet can be challenging, but there are several strategies to help you stay on track:

Education and Understanding: Learn as much as you can about your condition and the dietary guidelines. Understanding why certain foods are restricted or recommended can make it easier to adhere to the diet.

Meal Planning: Plan your meals. This helps ensure you have the right ingredients on hand and reduces the temptation to stray from your diet when hunger strikes.

Seek Professional Guidance: Work closely with a registered dietitian or a healthcare professional specializing in renal nutrition. They can provide personalized advice and meal plans tailored to your specific needs.

Portion Control: Pay attention to portion sizes. Even foods that are considered healthy can be problematic if consumed in large quantities. Use measuring cups or a food scale if needed.

Food Journaling: Keep a food diary to track what you eat and how it affects your health. This can help identify patterns and make necessary adjustments to your diet.

Gradual Changes: If the diet requires significant changes from your current eating habits, consider making gradual adjustments. It can be less overwhelming and easier to sustain in the long term.

Support System: Share your dietary goals with friends, family, or a support group. Having a support system can provide encouragement and accountability.

Explore Variety: Find creative ways to prepare meals within the dietary restrictions. Experiment with new recipes, flavors, and cooking methods to prevent boredom with the limited choices.

Healthy Substitutions: Identify and incorporate healthy substitutions for restricted foods. For example, replacing high-sodium seasonings with herbs and spices or choosing healthier cooking methods like baking or grilling instead of frying.

Stay Hydrated: Proper hydration is crucial for kidney health. Monitor your fluid intake as advised by your healthcare professional.

Manage Stress: Stress can impact eating habits. Find stress-relieving activities like meditation, yoga, or hobbies to help manage stress levels and avoid stress-induced eating.

Tips on tasty food without salt

Herbs and Spices: Experiment with various herbs and spices to add depth and complexity to your dishes. Use fresh herbs like parsley, basil, cilantro, or mint, and spices such as cumin, paprika, turmeric, and garlic powder to season your food.

Citrus Zest and Juice: Citrus fruits like lemons, limes, and oranges can bring brightness and tanginess to your meals. Use their zest and juice to enhance the flavor of salads, meats, and vegetables.

Vinegar: Balsamic, apple cider, and other flavored vinegar can add a pleasant acidity to dishes. Use them sparingly to avoid overpowering the flavors.

Onion and Garlic: These aromatic vegetables can significantly enhance the taste of your dishes. Experiment with sautéing or roasting them to bring out their natural sweetness.

Homemade Stocks and Broths: Make your stocks using herbs, vegetables, and bones (if allowed in your diet) to create a flavorful base for soups, stews, and sauces.

Herb Blends and Marinades: Create custom herb blends or marinades using a combination of your favorite spices, herbs, and acidic ingredients like vinegar or citrus juice to marinate meats and vegetables.

Umami-rich Ingredients: Incorporate umami-rich foods like mushrooms, tomatoes, and miso paste to add depth and savory flavors to your dishes.

Fresh Ingredients: Use fresh, high-quality ingredients to bring out natural flavors. Ripe tomatoes, sweet bell peppers, and other fresh produce can add sweetness and depth to your meals.

Avoid Pre-Packaged and Processed Foods: Processed foods often contain high amounts of sodium. opt for fresh, whole foods that you can season yourself.

MEASUREMENT CONVERSION CHART

1 teaspoon (tsp) = 5 milliliters (ml)

1 tablespoon (tbsp) = 3 teaspoons = 15 milliliters

1 fluid ounce = 2 tablespoons = 30 milliliters

1 cup = 8 fluid ounces = 16 tablespoons = 240 milliliters

1 pint = 2 cups = 16 fluid ounces = 480 milliliters

1 quart = 4 cups = 32 fluid ounces = 960 milliliters

1 gallon = 4 quarts = 16 cups = 128 fluid ounces = 3.8 liters

Weight Measurements:

1 ounce (oz) = 28.35 grams (g)

1 pound (lb.) = 16 ounces = 453.59 grams

1 kilogram (kg) = 2.205 pounds = 1000 grams

Common Kitchen Equivalents:

1 stick of butter = 1/2 cup = 113.4 grams

1 standard US cup of flour = 120 grams

1 standard US cup of granulated sugar = 200 grams

1 standard US cup of water = 240 milliliters = 240 grams

1 clove of garlic = approximately 1 teaspoon minced

7 weeks meal plan with a sample

MEAL PLAN WEEK 1

MONDAY
Breakfast: Egg white and veggie scramble
Lunch: baked cod with herbs
Dinner: veggie quinoa bowl
Snacks/ dessert: mango sorbet, roasted chickpea

TUESDAY
Breakfast: breakfast wrap with turkey and spinach
Lunch: turkey and bean chili
Dinner: ratatouille
Snacks/ dessert: coconut rice pudding, trail mix

WEDNESDAY
Breakfast: peanut butter and banana toast
Lunch: spinach feta chicken breast
Dinner: chicken and broccoli alfredo
Snacks/ dessert: date and walnut bars, carrot apple juice

THURSDAY
Breakfast: berries and millet porridge
Lunch: mushroom and spinach frittata
Dinner: shrimp and asparagus stir fry
Snacks/ dessert: gingerbread cookies, berry smoothie

FRIDAY
Breakfast: breakfast sausage patties
Lunch: cauliflower rice stir fry
Dinner: spaghetti squash and tomato sauce
Snacks/ dessert: baked sweet potato fries, watermelon slush

SATURDAY
Breakfast: pancakes
Lunch: roasted vegetable pasta
Dinner: veggie-packed turkey meatballs
Snacks/ dessert: lemon yogurt cake, yogurt parfait

SUNDAY
Breakfast: Greek yogurt parfait and seeds
Lunch: grilled lemon herb chicken
Dinner: veggie lentil curry
Snacks/ dessert: carrot cake muffins, cherry almond smoothie

MEAL PLAN WEEK 2
MONDAY
Breakfast:
Lunch:
Dinner:
Snacks/ dessert:

TUESDAY
Breakfast:
Lunch:
Dinner:
Snacks/ dessert:

WEDNESDAY
Breakfast:
Lunch:
Dinner:
Snacks/ dessert:

THURSDAY
Breakfast:

Lunch:
Dinner:
Snacks/ dessert:

FRIDAY
Breakfast:
Lunch:
Dinner:
Snacks/ dessert:

SATURDAY
Breakfast:
Lunch:
Dinner:
Snacks/ dessert:

SUNDAY
Breakfast:
Lunch:
Dinner:
Snacks/ dessert:

MEAL PLAN WEEK 3
MONDAY
Breakfast:
Lunch:
Dinner:
Snacks/ dessert:

TUESDAY
Breakfast:
Lunch:
Dinner:
Snacks/ dessert:

WEDNESDAY
Breakfast:
Lunch:
Dinner:
Snacks/ dessert:

THURSDAY
Breakfast:
Lunch:
Dinner:
Snacks/ dessert:

FRIDAY
Breakfast:
Lunch:
Dinner:
Snacks/ dessert:

SATURDAY
Breakfast:
Lunch:
Dinner:
Snacks/ dessert:

SUNDAY
Breakfast:
Lunch:
Dinner:
Snacks/ dessert:

MEAL PLAN WEEK 4
MONDAY
Breakfast:
Lunch:

Dinner:
Snacks/ dessert:

TUESDAY
Breakfast:
Lunch:
Dinner:
Snacks/ dessert:

WEDNESDAY
Breakfast:
Lunch:
Dinner:
Snacks/ dessert:

THURSDAY
Breakfast:
Lunch:
Dinner:
Snacks/ dessert:

FRIDAY
Breakfast:
Lunch:
Dinner:
Snacks/ dessert:

SATURDAY
Breakfast:
Lunch:
Dinner:
Snacks/ dessert:

SUNDAY

Breakfast:
Lunch:
Dinner:
Snacks/ dessert:

MEAL PLAN WEEK 5
MONDAY
Breakfast:
Lunch:
Dinner:
Snacks/ dessert:

TUESDAY
Breakfast:
Lunch:
Dinner:
Snacks/ dessert:

WEDNESDAY
Breakfast:
Lunch:
Dinner:
Snacks/ dessert:

THURSDAY
Breakfast:
Lunch:
Dinner:
Snacks/ dessert:

FRIDAY
Breakfast:
Lunch:
Dinner:

Snacks/ dessert:

SATURDAY
Breakfast:
Lunch:
Dinner:
Snacks/ dessert:

SUNDAY
Breakfast:
Lunch:
Dinner:
Snacks/ dessert:

MEAL PLAN WEEK 6

MONDAY

Breakfast:
Lunch:
Dinner:
Snacks/ dessert:

TUESDAY

Breakfast:
Lunch:
Dinner:
Snacks/ dessert:

WEDNESDAY

Breakfast:
Lunch:

Dinner:
Snacks/ dessert:

THURSDAY

Breakfast:
Lunch:
Dinner:
Snacks/ dessert:

FRIDAY

Breakfast:
Lunch:
Dinner:
Snacks/ dessert:

SATURDAY

Breakfast:
Lunch:
Dinner:
Snacks/ dessert:

SUNDAY

Breakfast:
Lunch:
Dinner:
Snacks/ dessert:

MEAL PLAN WEEK 7

MONDAY

Breakfast:

Lunch:
Dinner:
Snacks/ dessert:

TUESDAY

Breakfast:
Lunch:
Dinner:
Snacks/ dessert:

WEDNESDAY

Breakfast:
Lunch:
Dinner:
Snacks/ dessert:

THURSDAY

Breakfast:
Lunch:
Dinner:
Snacks/ dessert:

FRIDAY

Breakfast:
Lunch:
Dinner:
Snacks/ dessert:

SATURDAY

Breakfast:
Lunch:

Dinner:
Snacks/ dessert:

SUNDAY

Breakfast:
Lunch:
Dinner:
Snacks/ dessert:

CONCLUSION

Embracing a renal diet isn't just about restrictions; it's an opportunity to discover a world of delicious, nourishing meals crafted specifically to support kidney health.

This cookbook is more than a collection of recipes—it's a guide to culinary creativity within the boundaries of a renal diet by harnessing the power of flavors, innovative ingredient swaps, and mindful cooking techniques, this book empowers individuals to savor every bite while nurturing their well-being.

With these recipes, embark on a flavorful journey that redefines what it means to eat healthily, ensuring both satisfaction and vitality on every plate.

Embarking on a new dietary journey can undoubtedly be challenging, especially when faced with the complexities of managing renal health. However, please know that you are not alone on this path, and your commitment to embracing a renal-friendly diet is a powerful step towards a healthier and more vibrant life.

It's important to approach this journey with a sense of compassion for yourself. Adjusting to dietary changes may take time, and it's okay to have moments of difficulty. Remember that you are making choices that contribute to your well-being and the strength of your incredible spirit.

Embarking on a renal-friendly diet is a courageous choice. Celebrate each step, focus on what you can enjoy, and remember that progress, not perfection, is the goal. Nourish your body with love, lean on your support network, and see this journey as a testament to your strength. Your commitment to health is commendable—wishing you resilience and joy on this transformative path.

HAPPY COOKING!